POMPE DISEASE DIET COOKBOOK

Essential Recipes and Nutrition Strategies to Enhance Health, Strength, and Quality of Life

By

Sofia Andrews

TABLE OF CONTENTS

INTRODUCTION

Understanding Pompe Disease

Pompe disease, also known as Glycogen Storage Disease Type II, is a rare genetic disorder that affects the body's ability to break down glycogen, a stored form of sugar used for energy. This disease leads to an accumulation of glycogen in the muscles, impairing their function and causing a variety of symptoms ranging from muscle weakness and respiratory issues to more severe complications if left unmanaged. Living with Pompe disease can be challenging, but with the right knowledge, support, and lifestyle changes, individuals can improve their quality of life significantly.

Importance of Diet in Managing Pompe Disease

Diet plays a crucial role in managing Pompe disease. Proper nutrition can help alleviate symptoms, improve muscle function, and enhance overall health. While there is no cure for Pompe disease, dietary modifications can provide substantial benefits. A balanced diet rich in essential nutrients supports muscle maintenance, boosts energy levels, and aids in managing weight, which is vital for individuals with muscle-related disorders.

This cookbook is designed to be your comprehensive guide to navigating the dietary challenges posed by Pompe disease.

It offers a collection of delicious and nutritious recipes tailored to meet the specific needs of individuals with this condition. Our aim is to provide you with practical, easy-to-follow recipes that not only cater to your dietary requirements but also bring joy to your meals.

CHAPTER ONE

How This Cookbook Can Help "POMPE DISEASE DIET COOKBOOK: Delicious and Nutritious Recipes to Support Your Health Journey" is more than just a collection of recipes. It's a resource that empowers you with the knowledge to make informed dietary choices.

This is the very thing that you can anticipate from this book:

Comprehensive Nutrition Information: Learn about the key nutrients essential for managing Pompe disease, including proteins, healthy fats, vitamins, and minerals. Discover the foods that should be included in your diet and those to avoid.

Practical Tips for Meal Planning and **Preparation:** Get practical advice on how to plan and prepare meals that are both nutritious and satisfying. From batch cooking to grocery shopping, we've got you covered.

Variety of Delicious Recipes: Enjoy a diverse range of recipes that cater to different tastes and dietary needs.

From energizing breakfasts and nourishing lunches to hearty dinners and delightful desserts, this cookbook offers something for everyone.

Sample Meal Plans: Find inspiration with our sample meal plans that provide a structured approach to eating well. These plans are designed to help you stick to your dietary goals without feeling deprived. Supportive Strategies for Better Health: Beyond recipes, this book offers supportive strategies to help you maintain a healthy lifestyle. Learn how to stay motivated, adapt recipes to your preferences, and find resources for additional support.
Our goal is to make your health journey as smooth and enjoyable as possible.

We believe that eating well should be a delightful experience, not a chore. With the right tools and resources, you can take control of your diet and positively impact your health.

So, let's embark on this journey together. Turn the page and discover how delicious and nutritious eating can support your health and well-being. Welcome to the **"POMPE DISEASE DIET COOKBOOK"**—your partner in health and culinary exploration.

Understanding Pompe Disease
Overview of Pompe Disease

Pompe disease, also known as Glycogen Storage Disease Type II, is a rare genetic disorder that disrupts the body's ability to break down glycogen, a stored form of sugar used for energy. This disease is caused by mutations in the GAA gene, which leads to a deficiency or malfunction of the enzyme acid alpha-glucosidase. As a result, glycogen accumulates in the muscles, impairing their function and leading to a range of symptoms.

The severity and onset of Pompe disease can vary. Infantile-onset Pompe disease typically appears within the first few months of life and can cause significant muscle weakness, respiratory issues, and heart problems. Late-onset Pompe disease may present later in childhood, adolescence, or adulthood, often manifesting as progressive muscle weakness and respiratory difficulties. Early diagnosis and intervention are crucial in managing the disease and improving quality of life.

Importance of Diet in Managing Pompe Disease

Diet plays a pivotal role in managing Pompe disease. While there is no cure, proper nutrition can help alleviate symptoms, support muscle function, and enhance overall well-being.

A balanced diet tailored to the needs of individuals with Pompe disease can provide essential nutrients that promote muscle maintenance, boost energy levels, and help manage weight.

Key nutrients such as proteins, healthy fats, vitamins, and minerals are vital for those with Pompe disease. Proteins support muscle repair and growth, while healthy fats provide sustained energy.

 Vitamins and minerals, including calcium, vitamin D, and B vitamins, are crucial for bone health and energy metabolism. Avoiding foods high in refined sugars and unhealthy fats is equally important, as these can contribute to weight gain and exacerbate symptoms.

How This Cookbook Can Help
The "POMPE DISEASE DIET
COOKBOOK: Delicious and Nutritious Recipes to Support Your Health Journey" is designed to be a comprehensive guide to navigating the dietary challenges associated with Pompe disease. This cookbook offers practical, easy-to-follow recipes that cater to the specific nutritional needs of individuals with this condition, ensuring that meals are both delicious and beneficial.

This is the very thing that you can anticipate from this book:

Comprehensive Nutrition Information: Understand the key nutrients essential for managing Pompe disease, and learn which foods to include and avoid in your diet.
Practical Tips for Meal Planning and **Preparation:** Gain practical advice on meal planning and preparation, including tips on batch cooking, grocery shopping, and making nutritious choices.
Variety of Delicious Recipes: Enjoy a diverse range of recipes that cater to different tastes and dietary needs, from energizing

breakfasts and nourishing lunches to hearty dinners and delightful desserts.

Sample Meal Plans: Find inspiration with sample meal plans designed to help you stick to your dietary goals without feeling deprived.

Supportive Strategies for Better Health: Discover supportive strategies to help you maintain a healthy lifestyle, stay motivated, adapt recipes to your preferences, and find additional resources for support.

Our goal is to make your health journey as smooth and enjoyable as possible. We believe that eating well should be a delightful experience, not a chore. With the right tools and resources, you can take control of your diet and positively impact your health.

Let's embark on this journey together. Turn the page and discover how delicious and nutritious eating can support your health and well-being. Welcome to the "**POMPE DISEASE DIET COOKBOOK**"—your partner in health and culinary exploration.

CHAPTER TWO

Nutrition Essentials for Pompe Disease

Key Nutrients and Their Benefits

Proteins

Proteins are vital for muscle repair and growth. Individuals with Pompe disease often experience muscle weakness and degeneration, making protein intake crucial. High-quality protein sources include lean meats, fish, eggs, dairy products, legumes, and nuts.

Incorporating these into your diet helps maintain muscle mass and support overall health.

Healthy Fats

Healthy fats provide a sustained source of energy and are essential for hormone production and cell function. Omega-3 fatty acids, found in fatty fish (such as salmon and mackerel), flaxseeds, chia seeds, and walnuts, have anti-inflammatory properties that can benefit muscle health. Different wellsprings of sound fats incorporate avocados, olive oil, and nuts.

Vitamins and Minerals

Nutrients and minerals assume a urgent part in generally wellbeing and prosperity.

**Key nutrients for individuals with
Pompe disease include:**

Calcium and Vitamin D: Essential for
bone health and muscle function. Good
sources include dairy products, leafy greens,
fortified plant-based milks, and sunlight
exposure for vitamin D.

B Vitamins: Important for energy
metabolism and muscle function. Found in
whole grains, lean meats, eggs, dairy
products, and leafy greens.

Antioxidants: Help combat oxidative stress and support muscle health. Tracked down in organic products, vegetables, nuts, and seeds.

Carbohydrates

While managing carbohydrate intake is important, especially to avoid excessive glycogen buildup, including complex carbohydrates in your diet is essential for sustained energy. Opt for whole grains, vegetables, fruits, and legumes, which provide fiber and essential nutrients.

Foods to Include and Avoid

Foods to Include:

Lean Proteins: Chicken, turkey, fish, lean cuts of beef and pork, eggs, tofu, legumes, and dairy products.

Solid Fats: Avocados, olive oil, nuts, seeds, and greasy fish.

Whole Grains: Brown rice, quinoa, whole wheat bread and pasta, oats, and barley.

Fruits and Vegetables: A variety of colorful fruits and vegetables to ensure a wide range of vitamins, minerals, and antioxidants.

Dairy or Dairy Alternatives: Milk, yogurt, cheese, and fortified plant-based milks.

Foods to Avoid

Refined Sugars: Sugary snacks, sodas, and desserts that provide empty calories and can contribute to weight gain. Processed Foods: Foods high in unhealthy fats, sodium, and additives, such as fast food, processed meats, and pre-packaged snacks.

Excessive Salt: High-sodium foods can lead to fluid retention and hypertension.

Limit the intake of salty snacks, canned soups, and processed foods.

Tips for Meal Planning and Preparation Plan Ahead

Weekly Meal Planning: Plan your meals and snacks for the week to ensure you have all necessary ingredients and can stick to your dietary goals.

Clump Cooking: Plan bigger parts of feasts and freeze individual servings. This makes it easier to have nutritious meals ready when you're short on time.

Grocery List: Create a grocery list based on your meal plan to avoid impulse purchases and ensure you have all the ingredients you need.

Balanced Meals

Include a Variety of Foods: Aim to include a source of protein, healthy fat, and complex carbohydrates in each meal.

Portion Control: Be mindful of portion sizes to avoid overeating and to maintain a healthy weight.

Adapt Recipes

Modify Recipes: Adapt recipes to fit your dietary needs by substituting ingredients where necessary. For example, use whole grain pasta instead of refined pasta, or replace butter with olive oil.

Healthy Cooking Methods: Opt for grilling, baking, steaming, and sautéing instead of frying to reduce unhealthy fat intake.

Stay Hydrated

Drink Plenty of Water: Staying hydrated is essential for overall health.Mean to drink something like 8 glasses of water a day.

Limit Sugary Beverages: Avoid sugary drinks and opt for water, herbal teas, or infused water with fruits and herbs.

By focusing on these nutrition essentials and following practical tips for meal planning and preparation, you can effectively manage Pompe disease and support your health journey. The recipes in this cookbook are designed to incorporate these principles, making it easier for you to enjoy delicious, nutritious meals every day.

CHAPTER THREE

Breakfast Recipes

1. Berry Chia Seed Pudding

Description: This Berry Chia Seed Pudding is a refreshing and nutritious breakfast option. Packed with antioxidants, fiber, and omega-3 fatty acids, it's a great way to start your day with a burst of energy.

Prep Time: 10 minutes
Cook Time: 0 minutes (overnight chilling)
Servings: 2

Nutritional Information (per serving):

- Calories: 250
- Protein: 7g
- Fat: 12g
- Carbohydrates: 29g
- Fiber: 10g

Ingredients:

- 1/4 cup chia seeds
- 1 cup unsweetened almond milk
- 1 tablespoon honey or maple syrup
- 1/2 teaspoon vanilla extract
- 1 cup mixed berries (blueberries, raspberries, strawberries)

- Fresh mint leaves (optional, for garnish)

Preparation Instructions:

In a medium bowl, combine chia seeds, almond milk, honey (or maple syrup), and vanilla extract.

Stir well to mix, ensuring no chia seeds are clumped together.

Cover the bowl and refrigerate for the time being or for somewhere around 4 hours.

Before serving, stir the pudding again to ensure it's evenly mixed.

Divide the pudding into two servings, top with mixed berries and garnish with fresh mint leaves if desired.

2. Spinach and Mushroom Frittata

Description: This Spinach and Mushroom Frittata is a protein-rich, savory breakfast that's easy to make and full of flavor. It's perfect for a hearty start to your day.

Prep Time: 10 minutes

Cook Time: 20 minutes

Servings: 4

Nutritional Information (per serving):

- Calories: 180
- Protein: 12g
- Fat: 12g
- Carbohydrates: 6g
- Fiber: 2g

Ingredients:

- 6 large eggs
- 1/4 cup milk (dairy or plant-based)
- 1 cup fresh spinach, chopped
- 1/2 cup mushrooms, sliced
- 1/4 cup onion, finely chopped
- 1/4 cup shredded cheese (optional)
- 1 tablespoon olive oil
- Salt and pepper to taste

Preparation Instructions:

Preheat your oven to 350°F (175°C).

In a large bowl, whisk together the eggs and milk. Season with salt and pepper.

Heat olive oil in an oven-safe skillet over medium heat. Add onions and mushrooms, and sauté until soft, about 5 minutes.

Add spinach to the skillet and cook until wilted, about 2 minutes.

Pour the egg mixture over the vegetables in the skillet. If using cheese, sprinkle it on top.

Cook on the stovetop for about 5 minutes, until the edges begin to set.

Transfer the skillet to the preheated oven and bake for 10-15 minutes, until the frittata is fully set and lightly golden.

Allow to cool slightly before slicing and serving.

3. Quinoa Breakfast Bowl

Description: This Quinoa Breakfast Bowl is a nutrient-dense and satisfying meal. Quinoa provides a complete protein source, while the added fruits and nuts offer vitamins, minerals, and healthy fats.

Prep Time: 10 minutes
Cook Time: 15 minutes
Servings: 2

Nutritional Information (per serving):

- Calories: 300
- Protein: 10g

- Fat: 10g

- Carbohydrates: 45g

- Fiber: 8g

Ingredients:

- 1/2 cup quinoa

- 1 cup water or milk (dairy or plant-based

- 1 tablespoon honey or maple syrup

- 1/2 teaspoon cinnamon

- 1/2 cup mixed berries (blueberries, strawberries, raspberries)

- 1/4 cup sliced almonds or walnuts

- 1 tablespoon chia seeds (optional)

- Fresh mint leaves (optional, for garnish)

Preparation Instructions:

Rinse quinoa under cold water.

In a small saucepan, combine quinoa and water (or milk). Bring to a boil, then reduce heat to low, cover, and simmer for 12-15 minutes, or until the quinoa is cooked and water is absorbed.

Remove from heat and fluff with a fork. Stir in honey (or maple syrup) and cinnamon.

Divide the quinoa into two bowls. Top each with mixed berries, sliced almonds (or walnuts), and chia seeds.

Garnish with fresh mint leaves if desired and serve warm.

4. Avocado Toast with a Twist

Description: Avocado Toast with a Twist adds a flavorful upgrade to the classic version with a hint of lemon and a sprinkle of seeds. It's quick, nutritious, and perfect for busy mornings.

Prep Time: 5 minutes

Cook Time: 5 minutes

Servings: 2

Nutritional Information (per serving):

- Calories: 250
- Protein: 6g
- Fat: 18g
- Carbohydrates: 20g
- Fiber: 7g

Ingredients:

- 2 slices whole grain bread
- 1 ripe avocado
- 1/2 lemon, juiced
- 1 tablespoon sunflower seeds
- 1 tablespoon pumpkin seeds
- Salt and pepper to taste
- Red pepper flakes (optional)

Preparation Instructions:

Toast the slices of whole grain bread to your desired level of crispiness.

While the bread is toasting, cut the avocado in half, remove the pit, and scoop the flesh into a bowl.

Mash the avocado with a fork, adding lemon juice, salt, and pepper to taste.

Spread the mashed avocado evenly onto the toasted bread.

Sprinkle sunflower seeds and pumpkin seeds over the avocado.

Add a pinch of red pepper flakes if desired for a spicy kick.

Serve immediately and enjoy.

5. Greek Yogurt Parfait

Description: This Greek Yogurt Parfait is a delightful and nutritious breakfast that layers creamy yogurt with fresh fruits and crunchy granola. It's perfect for a quick and healthy start to your day.

Prep Time: 5 minutes

Cook Time: 0 minutes

Servings: 2

Nutritional Information (per serving):

- Calories: 200
- Protein: 12g
- Fat: 5g
- Carbohydrates: 28g
- Fiber: 4g

Ingredients:

- 1 cup Greek yogurt
- 1/2 cup granola (preferably low-sugar)

- 1 cup mixed berries (blueberries, strawberries, raspberries)
- 1 tablespoon honey or maple syrup
- Fresh mint leaves (optional, for garnish)

Preparation Instructions:

In two serving glasses or bowls, layer the ingredients starting with a few spoonfuls of Greek yogurt.

Add a layer of mixed berries, followed by a layer of granola.

Repeat the layers until all ingredients are used up.

Drizzle honey (or maple syrup) over the top.

Garnish with fresh mint leaves if desired.

Serve immediately and enjoy.

6. Oatmeal with Fruits and Nuts

Description: This Oatmeal with Fruits and Nuts is a warm, comforting breakfast packed with fiber, protein, and healthy fats. It's customizable and perfect for a nutritious start to your day.

Prep Time: 5 minutes
Cook Time: 10 minutes
Servings: 2

Nutritional Information (per serving):

- Calories: 300
- Protein: 8g
- Fat: 10g
- Carbohydrates: 45g

- Fiber: 8g

Ingredients:

- 1 cup rolled oats
- Cups water or milk (dairy or plant-based)
- 1 tablespoon honey or maple syrup
- 1/2 teaspoon cinnamon
- 1/2 cup mixed fresh fruits (such as banana slices, berries, apple chunks)
- 1/4 cup mixed nuts (such as almonds, walnuts, pecans)
- 1 tablespoon chia seeds or flaxseeds (optional)

Preparation Instructions:

In a medium saucepan, bring water (or milk) to a boil.

Stir in the rolled oats and reduce heat to medium-low.

Cook, stirring occasionally, until the oats are tender and the liquid is absorbed, about 5-7 minutes.

Remove from heat and stir in honey (or maple syrup) and cinnamon.

Divide the oatmeal into two bowls.

Top with mixed fresh fruits and nuts.

Sprinkle with chia seeds or flaxseeds if desired.

Serve warm and enjoy.

These breakfast recipes are designed to be both delicious and nutritious, providing the energy and nutrients needed to start your day off right.

Lunch Recipes

1. Grilled Chicken and Veggie Wrap
Description: This Grilled Chicken and Veggie Wrap is a balanced, protein-packed lunch option. Filled with lean chicken and colorful vegetables, it's both nutritious and satisfying.

Prep Time: 15 minutes
Cook Time: 15 minutes
Servings: 2

Nutritional Information (per serving):

- Calories: 350
- Protein: 25g
- Fat: 12g
- Carbohydrates: 35g
- Fiber: 6g

Ingredients:

- 2 boneless, skinless chicken breasts
- 1 tablespoon olive oil
- Salt and pepper to taste
- 1 teaspoon garlic powder
- 1 teaspoon paprika
- 1 red bell pepper, sliced
- 1 yellow bell pepper, sliced

- 1 small red onion, sliced
- 2 whole wheat tortillas
- 1/2 cup hummus
- Fresh spinach leaves

Preparation Instructions:

Preheat the grill to medium-high heat.

Brush chicken breasts with olive oil and season with salt, pepper, garlic powder, and paprika.

Grill the chicken for 6-7 minutes per side or until fully cooked. Let rest for a few minutes, then slice into strips.

While the chicken is grilling, sauté the bell peppers and onion in a skillet over medium heat until softened, about 5 minutes.

Spread hummus evenly over each tortilla.

Layer the spinach leaves, grilled chicken strips, and sautéed vegetables on top.
Roll up the tortillas tightly and slice in half to serve.

2. Lentil and Kale Salad

Description: This Lentil and Kale Salad is a nutrient-dense, fiber-rich lunch that is both filling and flavorful.
 The combination of lentils and kale provides a good source of protein, vitamins, and minerals.

Prep Time: 10 minutes
Cook Time: 20 minutes
Servings: 2

Nutritional Information (per serving):

- Calories: 300
- Protein: 15g
- Fat: 10g
- Carbohydrates: 40g
- Fiber: 15g

Ingredients:

- 1 cup cooked lentils
- 2 cups chopped kale
- 1/2 cup cherry tomatoes, halved
- 1/4 cup red onion, finely chopped

- 1/4 cup feta cheese, crumbled
- 2 tablespoons olive oil
- 1 tablespoon balsamic vinegar
- 1 teaspoon Dijon mustard
- Salt and pepper to taste

Preparation Instructions:

In a large bowl, combine cooked lentils, kale, cherry tomatoes, red onion, and feta cheese.

In a small bowl, whisk together olive oil, balsamic vinegar, Dijon mustard, salt, and pepper.

Pour the dressing over the salad and toss to combine.

Serve immediately or refrigerate until ready to eat.

3. Quinoa and Black Bean Salad

Description: This Quinoa and Black Bean Salad is a hearty and nutritious lunch option. It's packed with plant-based protein, fiber, and a variety of colorful vegetables.

Prep Time: 15 minutes
Cook Time: 15 minutes
Servings: 2

Nutritional Information (Ingredients:

- 1/2 cup quinoa
- 1 cup water
- 1 cup black beans, rinsed and drained
- 1/2 cup corn kernels
- 1/2 cup cherry tomatoes, halved

- 1/4 cup red bell pepper, diced
- 1/4 cup red onion, finely chopped
- 1/4 cup fresh cilantro, chopped
- 2 tablespoons olive oil
- 1 tablespoon lime juice
- 1/2 teaspoon cumin
- Salt and pepper to taste

Preparation Instructions:

Rinse quinoa under cold water.

In a small saucepan, bring water to a boil.

Add quinoa, reduce heat to low, cover, and simmer for 12-15 minutes, or until water is absorbed.

Remove from heat and let quinoa cool.

In a large bowl, combine cooked quinoa, black beans, corn, cherry tomatoes, red bell pepper, red onion, and cilantro.

In a small bowl, whisk together olive oil, lime juice, cumin, salt, and pepper.
Pour the dressing over the salad and toss to combine.
Serve immediately or refrigerate until ready to eat.

4. Tomato and Basil Soup

Description: This Tomato and Basil Soup is a comforting and healthy lunch option. Made with fresh tomatoes and aromatic basil, it's perfect for a light but satisfying meal.

Prep Time: 10 minutes

Cook Time: 30 minutes

Servings: 4

Nutritional Information (per serving):

- Calories: 150
- Protein: 4g
- Fat: 8g
- Carbohydrates: 18g
- Fiber: 4

Ingredients:
- 2 tablespoons olive oil
- 1 medium onion, chopped
- 2 cloves garlic, minced

- 6 large tomatoes, chopped

- 2 cups vegetable broth

- 1/4 cup fresh basil leaves, chopped

- Salt and pepper to taste

- 1/4 cup heavy cream or coconut milk (optional)

Preparation Instructions:

In a large pot, heat olive oil over medium heat. Add onion and garlic and sauté until softened, about 5 minutes.

Add chopped tomatoes and cook for another 10 minutes until they start to break down. Pour in the vegetable broth and bring to a boil. Reduce heat and simmer for 15 minutes.

Use an immersion blender to puree the soup
until smooth. Alternatively, transfer to a
blender in batches and blend until smooth.
Stir in chopped basil, salt, and pepper. If
desired, add heavy cream or coconut milk
for a creamier texture.
Serve hot, garnished with additional basil
leaves if desired.

5. Salmon and Asparagus Salad

Description: This Salmon and Asparagus
Salad is a light, protein-rich lunch that's
packed with omega-3 fatty acids, vitamins,
and minerals. It's perfect for a nutritious
and delicious meal.

Prep Time: 10 minutes

Cook Time: 20 minutes

Servings: 2

Nutritional Information (per serving):

- Calories: 350
- Protein: 25g
- Fat: 20g
- Carbohydrates: 10g
- Fiber: 4g

Ingredients:

- 2 salmon filets
- 1 tablespoon olive oil
- Salt and pepper to taste
- 1 bunch asparagus, trimmed
- 4 cups mixed greens

- 1/2 cup cherry tomatoes, halved
- 1/4 cup red onion, thinly sliced
- 2 tablespoons balsamic vinegar
- 1 tablespoon Dijon mustard
- 1 tablespoon honey
- 1/4 cup olive oil

Preparation Instructions:

Preheat the oven to 400°F (200°C).

Place salmon fillets on a baking sheet lined with parchment paper. Drizzle with olive oil and season with salt and pepper.

Bake for 15-20 minutes or until the salmon is cooked through.

While the salmon is baking, steam the asparagus until tender, about 5 minutes.

In a small bowl, whisk together balsamic vinegar, Dijon mustard, honey, and olive oil.

In a large bowl, combine mixed greens, cherry tomatoes, red onion, and steamed asparagus.

Flake the baked salmon into large pieces and add to the salad.

Drizzle with the balsamic dressing and toss to combine.

Serve immediately.

6. Turkey and Avocado Sandwich

Description: This Turkey and Avocado Sandwich is a quick, healthy, and delicious lunch option. It's filled with lean turkey, creamy avocado, and fresh vegetables for a satisfying meal.

Prep Time: 10 minutes

Cook Time: 0 minutes

Servings: 2

Nutritional Information (per serving):

- Calories: 350
- Protein: 20g
- Fat: 15g
- Carbohydrates: 35g
- Fiber: 7g

Ingredients:

- 4 slices whole grain bread

- 1/2 pound sliced turkey breast
- 1 ripe avocado, sliced
- 1 small tomato, sliced
- 1/2 cucumber, sliced
- 1/4 red onion, thinly sliced
- 2 tablespoons hummus
- Salt and pepper to taste

Preparation Instructions:

Toast the slices of whole grain bread if desired.

Spread hummus evenly on two slices of bread.

Layer the turkey, avocado, tomato, cucumber, and red onion on top of the hummus.

Season with salt and pepper to taste.

Top with the remaining slices of bread. Cut sandwiches in half and serve immediately.

These lunch recipes are designed to be both nutritious and delicious, providing the energy and nutrients needed to keep you going throughout the day.

Dinner Recipes

1. Baked Lemon Herb Salmon

Description: This Baked Lemon Herb Salmon is a flavorful and nutritious dinner option. The combination of lemon and herbs enhances the natural taste of the salmon while keeping it light and healthy.

Prep Time: 10 minutes
Cook Time: 20 minutes
Servings: 2

Nutritional Information (per serving):

- Calories: 350
- Protein: 30g
- Fat: 20g
- Carbohydrates: 5g
- Fiber: 1g

Preparation Instructions:

- 2 salmon filets
- 2 tablespoons olive oil

- 1 lemon, thinly sliced
- 2 cloves garlic, minced
- 1 tablespoon fresh dill, chopped
- 1 tablespoon fresh parsley, chopped
- Salt and pepper to taste.

Preparation Instructions:

Preheat the oven to 375°F (190°C).

Place salmon filets on a baking sheet lined with parchment paper.

Drizzle olive oil over the salmon and season with salt and pepper.

Top each filet with minced garlic, lemon slices, dill, and parsley.

Bake for 20 minutes, or until the salmon is cooked through and flakes easily with a fork.

Serve immediately with your favorite side dishes.

2. Quinoa-Stuffed Bell Peppers

Description: These Quinoa-Stuffed Bell Peppers are a colorful and nutrient-dense dinner. Packed with protein-rich quinoa, black beans, and vegetables, they make a filling and delicious meal.

Prep Time: 15 minutes
Cook Time: 30 minutes
Servings: 4

Nutritional Information (per serving):

- Calories: 250

- Protein: 10g
- Fat: 8g
- Carbohydrates: 35g
- Fiber: 10g

Ingredients:
- 4 large bell peppers (any color)
- 1 cup cooked quinoa
- 1 cup black beans, rinsed and drained
- 1/2 cup corn kernels
- 1/2 cup diced tomatoes
- 1/4 cup red onion, finely chopped
- 1 teaspoon cumin
- 1 teaspoon chili powder
- Salt and pepper to taste
- 1/2 cup shredded cheese (optional)
- Fresh cilantro for garnish

Preparation Instructions:

Preheat the oven to 375°F (190°C).

Cut the tops off the bell peppers and remove the seeds and membranes.

In a large bowl, combine cooked quinoa, black beans, corn, diced tomatoes, red onion, cumin, chili powder, salt, and pepper.

Stuff the bell peppers with the quinoa mixture and place them in a baking dish.

If using, sprinkle shredded cheese on top of each stuffed pepper.

Cover the dish with aluminum foil and bake for 25 minutes.

Remove the foil and bake for an additional 5 minutes, until the cheese is melted and bubbly.

Garnish with fresh cilantro and serve.

3. Garlic Butter Shrimp and Asparagus

Description: This Garlic Butter Shrimp and Asparagus dish is a quick and flavorful dinner option.

The combination of garlic, butter, and lemon creates a delicious sauce that pairs perfectly with shrimp and asparagus.

Prep Time: 10 minutes
Cook Time: 15 minutes
Servings: 2

Nutritional Information (per serving):

- Calories: 300
- Protein: 25g
- Fat: 18g
- Carbohydrates: 10g
- Fiber: 3g

Ingredients:

- 1 pound shrimp, peeled and deveined
- 1 bunch asparagus, trimmed and cut into 2-inch pieces
- 3 tablespoons butter

- 4 cloves garlic, minced
- 1 lemon, juiced
- Salt and pepper to taste
- Fresh parsley for garnish

Preparation Instructions:

In a large skillet, melt butter over medium heat.

Add garlic and cook until fragrant, about 1 minute.

Add shrimp and asparagus to the skillet, and season with salt and pepper.

Cook, stirring frequently, until the shrimp is pink and opaque, and the asparagus is tender, about 5-7 minutes.

Squeeze lemon juice over the shrimp and asparagus, and stir to combine.

Garnish with fresh parsley and serve immediately.

4. Chickpea and Spinach Curry

Description: This Chickpea and Spinach Curry is a hearty and nutritious vegan dinner option. It's packed with protein and fiber, and the spices add a delicious depth of flavor.

Prep Time: 10 minutes
Cook Time: 25 minutes
Servings: 4

Nutritional Information (per serving):

- Calories: 300
- Protein: 10g
- Fat: 12g
- Carbohydrates: 40g
- Fiber: 10g

Ingredients:

- 1 tablespoon olive oil
- 1 onion, finely chopped
- 3 cloves garlic, minced
- 1 tablespoon ginger, grated
- 1 tablespoon curry powder
- 1 teaspoon cumin
- 1/2 teaspoon turmeric
- 1/2 teaspoon cinnamon

- 1 can (15 oz) chickpeas, rinsed and drained
- 1 can (14 oz) diced tomatoes
- 1 can (14 oz) coconut milk
- 4 cups fresh spinach
- Salt and pepper to taste
- Fresh cilantro for garnish

Preparation Instructions:

In a large pot, heat olive oil over medium heat.

Add onion, garlic, and ginger, and sauté until the onion is translucent, about 5 minutes.

Add curry powder, cumin, turmeric, and cinnamon, and cook for another minute until fragrant.

Stir in chickpeas, diced tomatoes, and coconut milk. Bring to a boil, then reduce heat and simmer for 15 minutes.

Add spinach and cook until wilted, about 2 minutes.

Season with salt and pepper to taste.

Garnish with fresh cilantro and serve with rice or naan.

5. Baked Zucchini Boats

Description: These Baked Zucchini Boats are a low-carb, nutritious dinner option. Filled with a savory mixture of ground turkey, tomatoes, and herbs, they are both delicious and satisfying.

Prep Time: 15 minutes

Cook Time: 30 minutes

Servings: 4

Nutritional Information (per serving):

- Calories: 220
- Protein: 20g
- Fat: 10g
- Carbohydrates: 12g
- Fiber: 4g

Ingredients:

- 4 large zucchinis
- 1 tablespoon olive oil

- 1 pound ground turkey
- 1 small onion, chopped
- 2 cloves garlic, minced
- 1 can (14 oz) diced tomatoes
- 1 teaspoon Italian seasoning
- Salt and pepper to taste
- 1/2 cup shredded mozzarella cheese (optional)
- Fresh basil for garnish

Preparation Instructions:

Preheat the oven to 375°F (190°C).

Cut the zucchinis in half lengthwise and scoop out the seeds to create boats.

Place the zucchini halves on a baking sheet and drizzle with olive oil. Season with salt and pepper.

In a large skillet, cook the ground turkey over medium heat until browned. Add onion and garlic, and cook until softened.

Stir in diced tomatoes and Italian seasoning. Cook for another 5 minutes until the mixture is heated through.

Spoon the turkey mixture into the zucchini boats and top with shredded mozzarella cheese if desired.

Bake for 25-30 minutes until the zucchinis are tender and the cheese is melted and bubbly.

Garnish with fresh basil and serve.

6. Sweet Potato and Black Bean Tacos

Description: These Sweet Potato and Black Bean Tacos are a flavorful and healthy dinner option. The combination of roasted sweet potatoes and black beans makes for a satisfying and nutritious meal.

Prep Time: 15 minutes
Cook Time: 25 minutes
Servings: 4

Nutritional Information (per serving):

- Calories: 300
- Protein: 10g

- Fat: 10g
- Carbohydrates: 45g
- Fiber: 12

Ingredients:

- 2 large sweet potatoes, peeled and diced
- 1 tablespoon olive oil
- 1 teaspoon chili powder
- 1 teaspoon cumin
- Salt and pepper to taste
- 1 can (15 oz) black beans, rinsed and drained
- 8 small corn tortillas
- 1/4 cup red onion, finely chopped
- 1/4 cup fresh cilantro, chopped
- 1 lime, cut into wedges

- 1/2 cup crumbled feta cheese (optional)

Preparation Instructions:

Preheat the oven to 400°F (200°C).

Place the diced sweet potatoes on a baking sheet and drizzle with olive oil. Sprinkle it with chili powder, cumin, salt, and pepper. Toss to coat.

Roast in the oven for 20-25 minutes, or until the sweet potatoes are tender and lightly browned.

In a small saucepan, heat the black beans over low heat until warmed through. Warm the corn tortillas in a dry skillet over medium intensity.

CHAPTER FOUR

Snacks and Appetizers

1. Hummus and Veggie Platter

Description: This Hummus and Veggie Platter is a simple, healthy, and delicious appetizer. It's perfect for parties or as a quick snack, offering a variety of fresh vegetables and creamy hummus.

Prep Time: 10 minutes
Cook Time: 0 minutes
Servings: 4

Nutritional Information (per serving):

- Calories: 150
- Protein: 5g
- Fat: 8g
- Carbohydrates: 16g
- Fiber: 4g

Ingredients:

- 1 cup hummus
- 1 red bell pepper, sliced
- 1 yellow bell pepper, sliced
- 1 cucumber, sliced
- 1 cup cherry tomatoes
- 2 carrots, cut into sticks
- 1 small bunch of celery, cut into sticks

Preparation Instructions:

- Arrange the sliced vegetables on a large platter.
- Place the hummus in the center of the platter.
- Serve immediately, or cover and refrigerate until ready to serve.

2. Baked Sweet Potato Fries

Description: These Baked Sweet Potato Fries are a healthier alternative to regular fries. They are crispy on the outside, tender on the inside, and seasoned to perfection.

Prep Time: 10 minutes

Cook Time: 25 minutes

Servings: 4

Nutritional Information (per serving):

- Calories: 180
- Protein: 2g
- Fat: 6g
- Carbohydrates: 30g

Fiber: 4g

Ingredients:

- 2 large sweet potatoes, peeled and cut into fries
- 2 tablespoons olive oil
- 1 teaspoon paprika
- 1/2 teaspoon garlic powder
- Salt and pepper to taste

Preparation Instructions

Preheat the oven to 425°F (220°C).

Spread the fries in a single layer on a baking sheet lined with parchment paper.

Bake for 25 minutes, turning halfway through, until the fries are crispy and golden brown.

Serve immediately with your favorite dipping sauce.

3. Avocado Toast

Description: This Avocado Toast is a simple and nutritious snack. It's made with whole grain bread nd topped with creamy avocado, offering a perfect balance of healthy fats and fiber.

Prep Time: 5 minutes
Cook Time: 0 minutes
Servings: 2
Nutritional Information (per serving):

- Calories: 250
- Protein: 6g
- Fat: 16g
- Carbohydrates: 22g
- Fiber: 8g

Ingredients:

- 2 slices whole grain bread, toasted
- 1 ripe avocado
- Salt and pepper to taste
- 1 tablespoon lemon juice
- Optional toppings: cherry tomatoes, red pepper flakes, fresh herbs
- Preparation Instructions:

- Mash the avocado in a small bowl and season with salt, pepper, and lemon juice.
- Add any desired toppings.
- Serve immediately.

4. Greek Yogurt and Berry Parfait

Description: This Greek Yogurt and Berry Parfait is a refreshing and healthy snack. It's layered with protein-rich Greek yogurt, fresh berries, and a touch of honey.

Prep Time: 5 minutes
Cook Time: 0 minutes
Servings: 2

Nutritional Information (per serving):

- Calories: 150
- Protein: 10g
- Fat: 3g
- Carbohydrates: 25g
- Fiber: 4g

Ingredients:

- 1 cup Greek yogurt
- 1 cup mixed berries (strawberries, blueberries, raspberries)
- 2 tablespoons honey
- 2 tablespoons granola (optional)
- Preparation Instructions:
- In two glasses or bowls, layer Greek yogurt, mixed berries, and honey.
- Repeat the layers until all ingredients are used.
- Top with granola if desired.
- Serve immediately.

5. Caprese Skewers

Description: These Caprese Skewers are a delightful appetizer that combines fresh mozzarella, cherry tomatoes, and basil, drizzled with balsamic glaze.

Prep Time: 10 minutes
Cook Time: 0 minutes
Servings: 4

Nutritional Information (per serving):

- Calories: 100
- Protein: 5g
- Fat: 7g

- Carbohydrates: 4g
- Fiber: 1g

Ingredients:

- 20 cherry tomatoes
- 20 small fresh mozzarella balls
  (bocconcini)
- 20 fresh basil leaves
- 2 tablespoons balsamic glaze
- Salt and pepper to taste

Preparation Instructions:

On each skewer, alternate cherry tomatoes,
mozzarella balls, and basil leaves.
Arrange the skewers on a serving platter.

Drizzle with balsamic glaze and season with salt and pepper.

Serve immediately.

6. Veggie Spring Rolls

Description: These Veggie Spring Rolls are a light and refreshing appetizer filled with fresh vegetables and served with a tangy dipping sauce.

Prep Time: 15 minutes
Cook Time: 0 minutes
Servings: 4

Nutritional Information (per serving):

- Calories: 120
- Protein: 3g
- Fat: 2g
- Carbohydrates: 24g
- Fiber: 4g

Ingredients:

- 8 rice paper wrappers
- 1 cup shredded carrots
- 1 cup cucumber, julienned
- 1 cup red bell pepper, julienned
- 1 cup purple cabbage, thinly sliced
- 1/2 cup fresh mint leaves

- 1/2 cup fresh cilantro leaves
- 1/2 cup fresh basil leaves

Dipping Sauce:

- 1/4 cup soy sauce
- 1 tablespoon rice vinegar
- 1 tablespoon lime juice
- 1 teaspoon honey
- 1 teaspoon sesame oil
- 1 clove garlic, minced

Preparation Instructions:

- Prepare the dipping sauce by mixing soy sauce, rice vinegar, lime juice, honey, sesame oil, and minced garlic in a small bowl. Set aside.

- Dip each rice paper wrapper in warm water for about 5 seconds to soften.
- Lay the softened wrapper on a flat surface and place a small amount of each vegetable and fresh herbs in the center.
- Repeat with the remaining wrappers and filling.
- Serve the spring rolls with the dipping sauce.
- These snacks and appetizers are designed to be both healthy and delicious, providing a variety of flavors and nutrients to keep you satisfied.

Smoothies and Beverages

1. Green Detox Smoothie

Description: This Green Detox Smoothie is packed with leafy greens, fruits, and a hint of ginger, making it a refreshing and nutritious way to start your day.

Prep Time: 5 minutes
Cook Time: 0 minutes
Servings: 2

Nutritional Information (per serving):

- Calories: 180
- Protein: 3g
- Fat: 2g

- Carbohydrates: 40g

- Fiber: 8g

Ingredients:

- 1 cup spinach

- 1 cup kale

- 1 green apple, cored and chopped

- 1 banana

- 1/2 cucumber

- 1 tablespoon fresh ginger, grated

- 1 cup coconut water

- 1 tablespoon chia seeds

- Preparation Instructions:

- Add all ingredients to a blender.

- Blend until smooth.

- Pour into glasses and serve immediately.

2. Berry Blast Smoothie

Description: This Berry Blast Smoothie is a delicious and antioxidant-rich beverage made with a blend of mixed berries, yogurt, and a touch of honey.

Prep Time: 5 minutes
Cook Time: 0 minutes
Servings: 2

Nutritional Information (per serving):

- Calories: 200
- Protein: 8g
- Fat: 3g
- Carbohydrates: 38g
- Fiber: 6g

Ingredients:

- 1 cup mixed berries (strawberries, blueberries, raspberries)
- 1 banana
- 1/2 cup Greek yogurt
- 1 cup almond milk
- 1 tablespoon honey

Preparation Instructions:

Add all ingredients to a blender.

Blend until smooth.

Pour into glasses and serve immediately.

3. Tropical Mango Smoothie

Description: This Tropical Mango Smoothie is a refreshing and creamy drink, perfect for hot days. It combines mango, pineapple, and coconut milk for a taste of the tropics.

Prep Time: 5 minutes
Cook Time: 0 minutes
Servings: 2

Nutritional Information (per serving):

- Calories: 210
- Protein: 2g

- Fat: 6g
- Carbohydrates: 40g
- Fiber: 5g

Ingredients:

- 1 cup frozen mango chunks
- 1/2 cup frozen pineapple chunks
- 1 banana
- 1 cup coconut milk
- 1 tablespoon lime juice

Preparation Instructions:

Add all ingredients to a blender.

Blend until smooth.

Pour into glasses and serve immediately.

4. Peanut Butter Banana Smoothie

Description: This Peanut Butter Banana Smoothie is a creamy and satisfying beverage, perfect for a post-workout snack or a quick breakfast.

Prep Time: 5 minutes
Cook Time: 0 minutes
Servings: 2

Nutritional Information (per serving):

- Calories: 250
- Protein: 8g
- Fat: 10g
- Carbohydrates: 35g
- Fiber: 4g

Ingredients:

- 2 bananas
- 2 tablespoons peanut butter
- 1 cup almond milk
- 1 tablespoon honey
- 1/2 teaspoon vanilla extract
- Preparation Instructions:

- Add all ingredients to a blender.
- Blend until smooth.
- Pour into glasses and serve immediately.

5. Orange Carrot Ginger Juice

Description: This Orange Carrot Ginger Juice is a vibrant and invigorating drink, packed with vitamins and a zing of ginger.

Prep Time: 10 minutes

Cook Time: 0 minutes

Servings: 2

Nutritional Information (per serving):

- Calories: 120
- Protein: 2g
- Fat: 0g
- Carbohydrates: 30g
- Fiber: 4g

Ingredients:

- 2 large oranges, peeled
- 3 large carrots, peeled and chopped.
-
- 1-inch piece of ginger, peeled
- 1 cup water

Preparation Instructions:

- Add all ingredients to a blender.
- Blend until smooth.
- Strain through a fine mesh sieve or cheesecloth if desired.
- Pour into glasses and serve immediately.

6. Iced Green Tea with Mint

Description: This Iced Green Tea with Mint is a refreshing and hydrating beverage, perfect for a hot day. It's lightly sweetened and infused with fresh mint.

Prep Time: 5 minutes

Cook Time: 5 minutes (plus cooling time)

Servings: 4

Nutritional Information (per serving):

- Calories: 30
- Protein: 0g
- Fat: 0g
- Carbohydrates: 8g
- Fiber: 0g

Ingredients:

- Remove the tea bags and stir in honey until dissolved.
- Add fresh mint leaves and let the tea cool to room temperature.
- Strain out the mint leaves and pour the tea into a pitcher.
- Refrigerate until chilled.
- Serve over ice and garnish with lemon slices.

7. Golden Turmeric Latte

Description: This Golden Turmeric Latte is a warm, soothing beverage with anti-inflammatory properties. It's made with turmeric, ginger, and a touch of honey.

Prep Time: 5 minutes

Cook Time: 5 minutes

Servings: 2

Nutritional Information (per serving):

- Calories: 90
- Protein: 2g
- Fat: 4g
- Carbohydrates: 12g
- Fiber: 1g

Ingredients:

- 2 cups almond milk
- 1 teaspoon turmeric powder
- 1/2 teaspoon ground ginger
- 1 tablespoon honey
- 1/2 teaspoon cinnamon
- 1/4 teaspoon black pepper

Preparation Instructions:

- In a small saucepan, combine all ingredients.
- Heat over medium heat, whisking constantly, until warm and well combined.
- Pour into mugs and serve immediately.

8. Strawberry Basil Lemonade

Description: This Strawberry Basil Lemonade is a refreshing twist on the classic lemonade. It's infused with fresh strawberries and basil for a unique and delicious flavor.

Prep Time: 10 minutes
Cook Time: 0 minutes
Servings: 4

Nutritional Information (per serving):

- Calories: 70
- Protein: 1g
- Fat: 0g

- Carbohydrates: 18g
- Fiber: 2g

Ingredients:

- 1 cup fresh strawberries, hulled and sliced
- 1/4 cup fresh basil leaves
- 1/2 cup lemon juice (about 4 lemons)
- 1/4 cup honey
- 4 cups cold water
- Ice cubes

Preparation Instructions:

In a blender, puree the strawberries and basil with a little water until smooth.

Strain the mixture through a fine mesh sieve into a pitcher.

Add lemon juice, honey, and cold water. Stir until well combined.

Serve over ice and enjoy.

9. Mango Lassi

Description: This Mango Lassi is a creamy and refreshing Indian drink made with mango, yogurt, and a hint of cardamom.

Prep Time: 5 minutes
Cook Time: 0 minutes
Servings: 2

Nutritional Information (per serving):

- Calories: 160
- Protein: 5g
- Fat: 3g
- Carbohydrates: 30g
- Fiber: 2g

Ingredients:

- 1 cup ripe mango chunks
- 1 cup plain yogurt
- 1/2 cup milk
- 1 tablespoon honey
- 1/4 teaspoon ground cardamom

Preparation Instructions:

Add all ingredients to a blender.

Blend until smooth.

Pour into glasses and serve immediately.

10. Chia Seed Lemon Water

Description: This Chia Seed Lemon Water is a hydrating and nutrient-rich beverage. The chia seeds add a unique texture and a boost of omega-3 fatty acids.

Prep Time: 5 minutes

Cook Time: 0 minutes

Servings: 2

Nutritional Information (per serving):

- Calories: 50
- Protein: 1g
- Fat: 2g
- Carbohydrates: 6g
- Fiber: 4g

Ingredients:

- 2 cups water
- 1 tablespoon chia seeds
- 1 tablespoon lemon juice
- 1 teaspoon honey.

Preparation Instructions:

In a large glass or jar, combine water, chia seeds, lemon juice, and honey.

Stir well to combine.

Let sit for 10 minutes to allow the chia seeds to expand.

Stir again and serve immediately.

These smoothies and beverages are designed to be both refreshing and nutritious, offering a variety of flavors and health benefits to keep you hydrated and satisfied throughout the day.

Desserts

1. Chocolate Avocado Mousse

Description: This Chocolate Avocado Mousse is a rich and creamy dessert that's both healthy and indulgent. The avocado provides a smooth texture while adding healthy fats.

Prep Time: 10 minutes
Cook Time: 0 minutes
Servings: 4

Nutritional Information (per serving):

- Calories: 220
- Protein: 3g
- Fat: 18g

- Carbohydrates: 18g
- Fiber: 7g

Ingredients:
- 2 ripe avocados
- 1/4 cup unsweetened cocoa powder
- 1/4 cup honey or maple syrup
- 1/4 cup almond milk
- 1 teaspoon vanilla extract
- Pinch of salt
- Preparation Instructions:
- Cut avocados in half, remove the pit, and scoop out the flesh into a blender.
- Add cocoa powder, honey, almond milk, vanilla extract, and salt.
- Blend until smooth and creamy.

- Spoon into serving bowls and refrigerate for at least 30 minutes before serving.

2. Berry Chia Pudding

Description: This Berry Chia Pudding is a nutritious and delicious dessert, made with chia seeds and fresh berries. It's perfect for a light dessert or a healthy snack.

Prep Time: 5 minutes
Cook Time: 0 minutes (plus 2 hours chilling time)
Servings: 4

Nutritional Information (per serving):

- Calories: 150
- Protein: 4g
- Fat: 7g
- Carbohydrates: 19g
- Fiber: 8g

Ingredients:

- 1/2 cup chia seeds
- 2 cups almond milk
- 1/4 cup honey or maple syrup
- 1 teaspoon vanilla extract
- 1 cup mixed berries (strawberries, blueberries, raspberries)

Preparation Instructions:

In a bowl, combine chia seeds, almond milk, honey, and vanilla extract.

Stir well and let sit for 10 minutes.

Stir again to break up any clumps, then cover and refrigerate for at least 2 hours or overnight.

Before serving, top with mixed berries.

3. Baked Apple with Cinnamon

Description: These Baked Apples with Cinnamon are a warm and comforting dessert. The apples are baked to perfection and seasoned with cinnamon and a touch of honey.

Prep Time: 10 minutes

Cook Time: 30 minutes

Servings: 4

Nutritional Information (per serving):

- Calories: 120
- Protein: 0g
- Fat: 1g
- Carbohydrates: 31g
- Fiber: 5g

Ingredients:

- 4 large apples
- 4 teaspoons honey
- 1 teaspoon ground cinnamon
- 1/4 cup chopped walnuts (optional)

Preparation Instructions:

Preheat the oven to 350°F (175°C).

Core the apples and place them in a baking dish.

Fill each apple with 1 teaspoon of honey and a sprinkle of cinnamon.

Top with chopped walnuts if using.

Bake for 30 minutes, until the apples are tender.

Serve warm.

4. Coconut Rice Pudding

Description: This Coconut Rice Pudding is a creamy and fragrant dessert made with coconut milk and a touch of vanilla. It's perfect for a comforting treat.

Prep Time: 5 minutes

Cook Time: 25 minutes

Servings: 4

Nutritional Information (per serving):

- Calories: 220
- Protein: 3g
- Fat: 9g
- Carbohydrates: 32g
- Fiber: 1g

Ingredients:

- 1/2 cup jasmine rice
- 1 can (14 oz) coconut milk
- 1 cup water

- 1/4 cup honey or maple syrup
- 1 teaspoon vanilla extract
- Pinch of salt

Preparation Instructions:

In a medium saucepan, combine rice, coconut milk, water, honey, and salt. Bring to a boil over medium heat, then reduce to a simmer. Cook, stirring frequently, until the rice is tender and the pudding is thickened, about 25 minutes. Stir in vanilla extract. Serve warm or chilled.

5. Almond Butter Cookies

Description: These Almond Butter Cookies are a delicious and healthy alternative to traditional cookies. Made with almond butter and oats, they're both chewy and satisfying.

Prep Time: 10 minutes
Cook Time: 10 minutes
Servings: 12 cookies

Nutritional Information (per cookie):

- Calories: 120
- Protein: 3g
- Fat: 8g
- Carbohydrates: 10g
- Fiber: 2g

Ingredients:

- 1 cup almond butter
- 1/2 cup rolled oats
- 1/4 cup honey or maple syrup
- 1 teaspoon vanilla extract
- 1/2 teaspoon baking soda
- Pinch of salt

Preparation Instructions:

Preheat the oven to 350°F (175°C).

In a bowl, mix together almond butter, oats, honey, vanilla extract, baking soda, and salt until well combined.

Scoop tablespoon-sized balls of dough onto a baking sheet lined with parchment paper.

Flatten each ball slightly with a fork.

Bake for 10 minutes, until the edges are golden.

Let cool on the baking sheet for a few minutes before transferring to a wire rack to cool completely.

6. Lemon Blueberry Sorbet

Description: This Lemon Blueberry Sorbet is a refreshing and tangy dessert, perfect for a hot day. It's made with fresh blueberries and a splash of lemon juice.

Prep Time: 10 minutes

Cook Time: 0 minutes (plus 2 hours freezing time)

Servings: 4

Nutritional Information (per serving):

- Calories: 90
- Protein: 0g
- Fat: 0g
- Carbohydrates: 22g
- Fiber: 3g

Ingredients:

- 2 cups fresh blueberries
- 1/2 cup water
- 1/4 cup honey or maple syrup
- 1/4 cup lemon juice

Preparation Instructions:

In a blender, combine blueberries, water, honey, and lemon juice.

Blend until smooth.

Pour the mixture into a shallow dish and freeze for 2 hours, stirring every 30 minutes.

Scoop into bowls and serve immediately.

7. Banana Nice Cream

Description: This Banana Nice Cream is a healthy and creamy alternative to ice cream. Made with just bananas and a splash of vanilla, it's both simple and delicious.

Prep Time: 5 minutes

Cook Time: 0 minutes (plus freezing time)

Servings: 4

Nutritional Information (per serving):

- Calories: 100
- Protein: 1g
- Fat: 0g
- Carbohydrates: 27g
- Fiber: 3g

Ingredients:

- 4 ripe bananas, sliced and frozen
- 1 teaspoon vanilla extract
- Preparation Instructions:
-
- Place the frozen banana slices in a blender or food processor.

- Blend until smooth, scraping down the sides as needed.
- Add vanilla extract and blend again.
- Serve immediately or freeze for an additional 30 minutes for a firmer texture.

8. Chocolate Dipped Strawberries

Description: These Chocolate Dipped Strawberries are a simple yet elegant dessert. They combine the sweetness of strawberries with the richness of dark chocolate.

Prep Time: 10 minutes

Cook Time: 5 minutes

Servings: 4

Nutritional Information (per serving):

- Calories: 150
- Protein: 2g
- Fat: 9g
- Carbohydrates: 18g
- Fiber: 4g

Ingredients:

- 1 pint fresh strawberries, washed and dried
- 1/2 cup dark chocolate chips
- 1 tablespoon coconut oil

Preparation Instructions:

In a microwave-safe bowl, combine dark chocolate chips and coconut oil.

Microwave in 30-second intervals, stirring after each, until fully melted and smooth.

Dip each strawberry into the melted chocolate, allowing excess to drip off.

Place on a parchment-lined baking sheet.

Serve chilled.

9. No-Bake Energy Bites

Description: These No-Bake Energy Bites are a quick and easy treat that's both healthy and satisfying. Made with oats, peanut butter, and honey, they are perfect for a quick snack or dessert.

Prep Time: 10 minutes
Cook Time: 0 minutes
Servings: 12 bites

Nutritional Information (per bite):

- Calories: 100
- Protein: 3g
- Fat: 5g
- Carbohydrates: 12g
- Fiber: 2g

Ingredients:

- 1 cup rolled oats
- 1/2 cup peanut butter
- 1/4 cup honey
- 1/4 cup flaxseed meal
- 1/4 cup chocolate chips
- 1 teaspoon vanilla extract

Preparation Instructions:

In a large bowl, combine all ingredients.

Mix well until thoroughly combined.

Roll the mixture into tablespoon-sized balls.

Refrigerate for at least 30 minutes before serving.

10. Spiced Apple Crumble

Description: This Spiced Apple Crumble is a warm and comforting dessert with a crunchy oat topping. It's perfect for a cozy evening treat.

Prep Time: 15 minutes
Cook Time: 30 minutes
Servings: 4

Nutritional Information (per serving):

- Calories: 250
- Protein: 3g
- Fat: 10g
- Carbohydrates: 40g
- Fiber: 5g

Ingredients:

- 4 large apples, peeled, cored, and sliced
- 1/4 cup honey or maple syrup
- 1 teaspoon ground cinnamon
- 1/2 teaspoon ground nutmeg
- 1 cup rolled oats
- 1/4 cup almond flour
- 1/4 cup coconut oil, melted

Preparation Instructions:

Preheat the oven to 350°F (175°C).

In a bowl, toss apple slices with honey, cinnamon, and nutmeg.

Spread the apples evenly in a baking dish.

In a separate bowl, combine oats, almond flour, and melted coconut oil.

Sprinkle the oat mixture over the apples.

Bake for 30 minutes, until the topping is golden and the apples are tender.

Serve warm.

These desserts offer a range of flavors and textures, providing delicious options that align with a healthy diet for managing Pompe disease.

CHAPTER FIVE

Meal Plans and Tips

Day 1:

Breakfast: Green Detox Smoothie

Lunch: Quinoa Salad with Grilled Chicken

Dinner: Baked Salmon with Steamed
Vegetables

Snack: Apple slices with almond butter

Day 2:

Breakfast: Berry Chia Pudding

Lunch: Lentil Soup with Whole Grain
Bread

Dinner: Turkey Meatballs with Zucchini
Noodles

Snack: Greek yogurt with mixed berries

Day 3:

Breakfast: Mango Lassi

Lunch: Chickpea Salad with Lemon Dressing

Dinner: Stir-Fried Tofu with Brown Rice

Snack: Carrot sticks with hummus

Day 4:

Breakfast: Peanut Butter Banana Smoothie

Lunch: Quinoa Stuffed Bell Peppers

Dinner: Grilled Chicken with Quinoa and Roasted Vegetables

Snack: Mixed nuts and dried fruits

Day 5:

Breakfast: Tropical Mango Smoothie

Lunch: Greek Salad with Grilled Shrimp

Dinner: Vegetable Stir-Fry with Tofu

Snack: Sliced cucumber with guacamole

Day 6:

Breakfast: Overnight Oats with Berries

Lunch: Sweet Potato and Black Bean Salad

Dinner: Baked Cod with Quinoa Pilaf

Snack: Rice cakes with almond butter

Day 7:

Breakfast: Green Smoothie Bowl with Granola

Lunch: Spinach and Feta Stuffed Chicken Breast

Dinner: Lentil Curry with Brown Rice

Snack: Fresh fruit salad

Tips for Sticking to Your Diet

Prepare: Invest energy every week arranging your dinners and snacks to stay away from drive eating.

Keep Healthy Snacks Handy: Stock up on nutritious snacks like fruits, nuts, and yogurt to curb cravings.

Remain Hydrated: Drink a lot of water over the course of the day to remain hydrated and keep up with energy levels.

Include Variety: Experiment with different recipes and ingredients to keep meals interesting and enjoyable.

Practice Portion Control: Use smaller plates and bowls to help control portion sizes.

Stand by listening to Your Body: Focus on craving and completion prompts to abstain from indulging.

Seek Support: Connect with others who share your dietary goals for motivation and encouragement.

Grocery Shopping List

Produce:

- Spinach
- Kale
- Mixed berries (strawberries, blueberries, raspberries)
- Bananas
- Apples
- Oranges
- Lemons
- Avocados
- Cucumber
- Bell peppers
- Carrots
- Sweet potatoes

Proteins:

- Chicken breast
- Turkey meatballs
- Salmon fillets
- Tofu
- Lentils
- Chickpeas
- Shrimp

Grains and Legumes:

- Quinoa
- Brown rice
- Whole grain bread
- Rolled oats

Dairy and Alternatives:

- Greek yogurt
- Almond milk
- Feta cheese (optional)

Nuts and Seeds:

- Almond butter
- Chia seeds
- Flaxseed meal
- Mixed nuts

Pantry Staples:

- Olive oil
- Coconut oil
- Honey
- Maple syrup

- Spices (cinnamon, ginger, nutmeg, turmeric)
- Vegetable broth

Frozen:
- Frozen mango chunks
- Frozen pineapple chunks
- Batch Cooking and Freezing Tips

Plan Ahead: Choose recipes that freeze well, such as soups, stews, and casseroles. Use Freezer-Friendly Containers: Invest in freezer-safe containers or resealable bags for storing meals.

Label and Date: Always label containers with the contents and date of preparation for easy identification.

Portion Control: Freeze meals in individual portions to avoid thawing more than needed.

Thaw Properly: Thaw frozen meals in the refrigerator overnight or use the defrost setting on your microwave.

Reheat Safely: Reheat frozen meals thoroughly to ensure they reach a safe internal temperature before consuming.

These meal plans and tips are designed to help you maintain a nutritious diet while managing Pompe disease, offering variety and practical strategies for success.

CONCLUSION

Your Health Journey

Your journey with Pompe disease is unique and requires dedication to managing your health through nutrition and lifestyle choices. By prioritizing your well-being and making informed dietary decisions, you can enhance your quality of life and overall health.

Staying Motivated

Maintaining motivation is key to successfully managing Pompe disease. Surround yourself with supportive friends, family, and healthcare professionals who understand your journey and can offer encouragement and guidance along the way.Keep in mind, each little step figures in with a better you.

Adapting Recipes to Your Preferences
The recipes in this cookbook are designed to be versatile and adaptable to your personal preferences and dietary needs. Feel free to experiment with ingredients and flavors to create meals that you enjoy while supporting your health goals.

Final Thoughts and Encouragement
Living with Pompe disease presents challenges, but it also offers opportunities for growth and resilience. Embrace each day with positivity and determination, knowing that you have the strength to overcome

obstacles and thrive. Stay informed, stay active, and celebrate your successes, big and small.